GLUCOSE REVOLT

COOKBOOK AND MEAL PLANS FOR ALL TYPES OF DIABETES

DR. JOHN A POWELL

Table of Contents

INTRODUCTION 5

CHAPTER ONE 6

  TYPE ONE DIABETES 6

  SYMPTOMS OF TYPE ONE DIABETES 8

  CAUSES OF TYPE ONE DIABETES 9

CHAPTER TWO 10

  TYPE 2 DIABETES 10

  SYMPTOMS OF TYPE 2 DIABETES 11

  CAUSES OF TYPE TWO DIABETES 13

  Other causes of type 2 diabetes 13

CHAPTER THREE 14

  GESTATIONAL DIABETES..14

  SYMPTOMS OF GESTATIONAL DIABETES 15

  CAUSES OF GESTATIONAL DIABETES 17

CHAPTER FOUR 18

  FOOD TO EAT OR AVOID (TYPE ONE DIABETES) 18

CHAPTER FIVE 21

  FOOD TO EAT OR AVOID (TYPE TWO DIABETES)..............21

CHAPTER SIX 30

  FOOD TO EAT OR AVOID (GESTATIONAL DIABETES) 30

CHAPTER SEVEN...34

  MEAL PLAN FOR TYPE ONE DIABETES 34

CHAPTER EIGHT 36

  MEAL PLAN FOR TYPE TWO DIABETES....................36

CHAPTER NINE...41

   MEAL PLAN FOR GESTATIONAL DIABETES.....................41

CHAPTER TEN..43

   RECIPES FOR TYPE ONE DIABETES.................................43

CHAPTER ELEVEN..47

   RECIPES FOR TYPE TWO DIABETES...............................47

CHAPTER TWELVE...74

   RECIPES FOR GESTATIONAL DIABETES..........................74

CHAPTER THIRTEEN..87

   CONCLUSION..87

INTRODUCTION

Diabetes may be a habitual complaint that happens either when the pancreas doesn't produce enough insulin or when the body can't effectively use the insulin it produces. Insulin may be a hormone that regulates blood sugar.

Hyperglycemia, also called raised blood sugar or raised blood glucose, may be a common effect of uncontrolled diabetes and over time results in serious damage to several of the body's systems, especially the jitters and blood vessels. In of grown- ups progressed 18 times and aged had diabetes.

In 2019, diabetes was the direct explanation for1.5 million deaths and 48 of all deaths thanks to diabetes passed before the age of 70 times. Another 460 000 renal complaint deaths were caused by diabetes, and raised blood sugar causes around 20 of cardiovascular deaths.   Between 2000 and 2019, there was a third increase in age- homogenized mortality rates from diabetes. In lower- middle- income countries, the death rate thanks to diabetes increased 13. By distinction, the probability of dying from anybody of the four main noninfectious conditions (cardiovascular conditions, cancer, habitual respiratory conditions or diabetes) between the ages of 30 and 70 dropped by 22 encyclopedically within 2000 and 2019.

CHAPTER ONE

TYPE ONE DIABETES

Type 1 diabetes is insulin deficiency and accounts for only 5% to 10% of all diabetics. Type 1 diabetes is more serious, but type 1 diabetes is less common. Type 1 diabetes is often referred to as juvenile diabetes, although type 1 diabetes can develop at any age, it is more common in childhood.

Explanation of Insulin:

Your blood has food (carbohydrates (or sugar)), oxygen, poisons, and toxins. Blood is where your cells get rid of waste products, but it's also where your cells get nutrients and oxygen. To avoid eating and dying, your body has set up a system that your cells need to look for only one digestive hormone: insulin. This alleviates a lot of the complex work that each cell has to do, allowing cells to find food (sugars) for their cells by simply relying on insulin.

All insulin does is transmit hormonal messages between sugar molecules (carbohydrates) and cells, enabling cells to find sugar in the blood and eat it. Yes, many contain various types of vitamins and nutrients, and others contain no vitamins and nutrients. It exists to handle complex disruptions. Also, not all cells receive all sugar molecules. Insulin ensures that sugars, including certain vitamins and nutrients, reach the right cells. Not all cells receive all sugar vitamins as nutrients. Vitamins are often dedicated to specific cells.

Instead of insulin itself lowering blood sugar levels, cells eat sugar to lower blood sugar levels, but cells cannot find sugar without the help of insulin.

When a cell receives a hormonal message to eat sugars attached to the cell's outer surface, the cell takes the sugar molecule into its mitochondria and, with the help of another enzyme, binds it to oxygen for energy. to chemically vibrate mitochondria. The chemical vibrations of mitochondria keep cells alive. If that sugar molecule contains some kind of vitamin or nutrient, then that vitamin or nutrient transfers that energy through a series of complex chemical chain reactions triggered by that burst of energy to literally perform functional work within that cell.

Sugars in fruits and vegetables always contain certain vitamins and nutrients. Refined sugar is not. Eating refined sugar is like running a car on gasoline without gear oil, the heating may work but the car is going nowhere and does nothing important. Producing that energy is a huge waste of insulin, enzymes and oxygen.

Explanation of Glucagon:

In type 1 diabetes, not only is the production of insulin damaged or destroyed, but the hormone glucagon is also damaged or destroyed. Glucagon is another important hormone produced by the pancreas when it detects low sugar levels. Digestive hormone. This hormone sends a message to the liver to produce more sugar from the fat stored in the body. If this hormone is not produced, the liver cannot receive the message and blood sugar levels are dangerous. Too low blood sugar can kill you, just like too low oxygen levels. Remember that without sugar you cannot metabolize oxygen. And those who cannot metabolize oxygen are called dead. For this reason, people with type 1 diabetes may also get an emergency injection of glucagon if they are unable to eat or buy sugar pills, candy, or fruit during hypo. What happens when the brain is deprived of sugar? In fact, at first, the brain is functioning and the victim cannot eat or drink anything.

SYMPTOMS OF TYPE ONE DIABETES

One of the most common indicators of type 1 diabetes is family history. Studies have shown that type 1 diabetes may also be associated with genetic and possibly viral causes. However, if you have a family history of type 1 diabetes, it's important to get regular screenings and tests, even if you don't have other symptoms. By diagnosing the disease early, you can better adapt to diet, lifestyle, and medication changes before it becomes severe enough to require more drastic measures.

Unfortunately, after being completely asymptomatic for most of life, type 1 diabetes can suddenly show unexpected symptoms. This can have a huge impact on a person's life, but recognizing the symptoms can help you know when medical attention is needed for diagnosis. If any of the following symptoms appear regularly, talk to your doctor about additional tests to determine if diabetes is the cause:

- Continually thirsty
- Frequent urination
- Increase in appetite accompanied by weight loss
- Fatigue
- Weakness
- Mood swings
- Irritability
- Vision problems
- Gastrointestinal issues
- Tests indicating high levels of sugar in blood or urine

The above symptoms are certainly indicative and common symptoms of type 1 diabetes. However, all symptoms can also be attributed to other diseases and conditions. For this reason, it is important to consult a doctor consciously and conscientiously. If you have symptoms and have a family history of diabetes, that should be a particularly strong indication that you may need an evaluation.

Early diagnosis and treatment are essential for managing type 1 diabetes. Insulin injections may be prescribed to maintain adequate insulin levels. You may also need to make changes in your diet and lifestyle. The sooner this is started, the better the patient will be. So, keep an eye on indicators and common symptoms, and get tested regularly if you have a family history of diabetes.

CAUSES OF TYPE ONE DIABETES

It's a common myth that eating too much sugar can lead to diabetes. This is a completely false belief. Your body needs sugar to metabolize oxygen. In fact, the only reason you're breathing oxygen right now is because you live for sugar. If you don't need sugar for energy, you don't need oxygen to live. Inability to metabolize sugar is a symptom of the disease, not the root cause. Sugar does not cause diabetes any more than oxygen causes lung cancer.

IMMUNE RESPONSE DISORDER is the primary cause of type 1 diabetes. Most of her Type 1 diabetics get sick about two weeks after recovering from serious illnesses like measles, flu, and food poisoning. Your immune system attacks and kills the islet cells in your pancreas simply because they happen to have a common antigen code that matches the antibodies your immune system produces, and the invading viruses. Type 1 diabetes may therefore be caused by a defective immune system that kills insulin-producing islet cells in the pancreas. But quite often also kills the islet cells that also produce the Digestive Hormone Glucagon as well.

CHAPTER TWO

TYPE 2 DIABETES

Type 2 diabetes, also called non-insulin dependent diabetes, is not related to insulin production in the body. Type 2 diabetes is caused by a condition known as insulin resistance. In this state insulin has failed to do its job of opening glucose channels into the cell and jumps when glucose molecules cannot enter the cell for use or storage. Blood flow back to cells can lead to high blood sugar levels or hyperglycemia.

So, what causes insulin resistance? In fact, most doctors and medical professionals cannot give an exact explanation for this. Usually they tend to answer this question vaguely in medical terms. So, the patient is no longer bothered by this question. Some of them tend to blame genetic or DNA-related problems. This is the most common "training answer" scientists give when they can't pinpoint the root cause of a disease.

This is a logical and easy-to-understand explanation (from a naturopathic perspective) of what actually causes insulin resistance. Type 2 diabetes is already a global threat to modern society, but it's not as complicated as it sounds. It doesn't take rocket science to explain why, and it doesn't need all those high-tech chemicals to overturn it.

Everyone knows that diabetes is a lifestyle disease. It's directly related to what you put in your mouth, but how? All this time, we are all blaming high-calorie, fatty, and sugary foods as the cause of the global diabetes pandemic. The first thing that comes to mind as soon as someone is diagnosed with diabetes is that simply reducing or eliminating sugary foods will cure the problem. Many diabetics follow this advice, but have their insulin resistance problems gone? No!

They have turned the picture upside down. Insulin resistance causes elevated blood sugar levels, not the result of hyperglycemia. Reducing your sugar intake won't address the root of the problem. It just makes you tired and lacks energy. The problem isn't having too much sugar. The problem is that the body's cells cannot utilize the glucose supply.

SYMPTOMS OF TYPE 2 DIABETES

Symptoms of type 2 diabetes usually develop gradually. Because of this, you may have been in this state for quite some time without knowing it. Seek immediate medical attention if any of the following signs or symptoms occur:

Increased thirst:

With so much glucose accumulating in your bloodstream, your body's tissues become dehydrated and you think you're thirsty.

Increased hunger:

With no insulin available in your system, your cells are unable to take in glucose and energy is drained out of your body's organs and muscle tissue. This can leave you very hungry.

Frequent urination:

Because of increased thirst, people may be able to drink more fluids than usual, resulting in more frequent urination.

Weight loss:

Despite the fact that you are still eating more because of your increased appetite, you can still lose weight. If your system cannot metabolize glucose, it uses alternative energy stored in muscle tissue and body fat., thereby burning calories.

Blurred eyesight:

If your blood sugar is too high, it can draw fluid out of your eye lens and affect your ability to concentrate.

Sections of discolored skin:

Some people with type 2 diabetes also create areas of darker, velvety skin, usually in the creases and folds of the body in the armpits and back of the neck. This problem is known as acanthosis and is also an indicator of insulin resistance.

Exhaustion:

When cells are deprived of glucose, they become extremely tired and sometimes grumpy at the same time.

Slow-healing wounds:

Type 2 diabetes affects the body's ability to repair itself.

Frequent infection:

This condition also affects your immune system's ability to fight infections, so you may get infected more often than usual.

If your doctor suspects you have type 2 diabetes, he or she will likely advise you to undergo several blood glucoses tests to determine if you have elevated glucose levels in your blood.

CAUSES OF TYPE TWO DIABETES

Type 2 diabetes can be described as a lifestyle disease, but it is primarily caused by two interrelated problems:

- ➤ The pancreas cannot produce enough insulin to control blood sugar levels in the body.

- ➤ Liver, fat, and muscle cells develop resistance to insulin due to abnormal cellular interactions with insulin, impairing the cells' ability to regulate sugar levels.

Other causes of type 2 diabetes

Aside from your body's inability to respond to insulin, other external factors can cause type 2 diabetes:

- ➤ Bad eating habits
- ➤ Overweight or living with obesity
- ➤ Lack of adequate physical activity and exercise
- ➤ Genetics – if someone else in the family has her type 2 diabetes

CHAPTER THREE

GESTATIONAL DIABETES

Gestational diabetes is diabetes that develops for the first time in a woman during pregnancy. Gestational diabetes goes away after the baby is born, but it puts you at an increased risk of developing diabetes later in life. Any type of diabetes during pregnancy increases the risk of problems for both baby and mother.

Pregnant women with gestational diabetes tend to have larger babies at birth. This increases the chances of problems during delivery. This fact should alert pregnant women and their doctors to encourage careful evaluation, diagnosis, and prompt treatment of women with gestational diabetes. Values should be monitored and controlled on a regular basis.

SYMPTOMS OF GESTATIONAL DIABETES

Women who are pregnant and have higher than normal blood sugar levels suffer from a condition known as gestational diabetes. The cause of this particular form of diabetes is unknown, but doctors and scientists believe it is related to the extra stress that pregnancy puts on a woman's body. Most women are asymptomatic. That is, they do not have symptoms of gestational diabetes and are unaware that they can contract this dangerous disease during pregnancy.

The placenta, the life support system of the fetus, is believed to be the underlying cause of the condition. It produces a variety of hormones during pregnancy, and some of these hormones alter the effectiveness of maternal insulin. Insulin's main job is to move glucose (sugar) from the bloodstream into cells for energy. is to When this is neglected, blood sugar levels rise and the body responds by producing more insulin. Often up to three times the normal amount. This is known as insulin resistance.

When a woman has signs and symptoms of gestational diabetes, it's usually a more familiar type that affects all people with diabetes, including:

> Frequent urination due to hyperglycemia.
> Being extremely thirsty all the time because of the increased urination.
> Extreme hunger caused by the inability of insulin to move sugar into cells. Even if there is enough sugar in the bloodstream, cells cannot use it, causing hunger.
> Weight loss because your body breaks down protein and fat when you think you're hungry.
> Fatigue as a result of an energy decrease.
> Blurred vision due to swelling of the lens due to increased blood volume.
> More irritability and moodiness.

As mentioned above, most women show no signs of gestational diabetes. This is why it is so important that all women between 24 and 28 weeks pregnant are screened for this condition.

The test used is an oral glucose tolerance test in which women drink a drink containing 50 g of concentrated glucose. Blood is drawn twice before and 1 hour after drinking the glucose drink. If her blood sugar is above 130-140 mg/dl she should have further tests done.

This is known as a 3-hour 100 g oral glucose tolerance test starting 3 days before blood sampling. During these three days, the woman eats as much as she pleases and per day, she consumes over 150 g of carbohydrates. The night before the test she stops eating at least 12 hours before her and in the morning, she drinks 100 g of glucose solution. Afterwards, she had blood drawn once before she drank glucose and then at 1-hour intervals for a total of four blood samples. Blood glucose levels should not exceed the following values for 2 or more tests:

- Fasting - 95mg/dl
- 1 hour - 180mg/dl
- 2 hours - 155mg/dl
- 3 hours - 140mg/dl

If there are no symptoms of gestational diabetes and the diagnosis is made based on test results, pregnant women should begin the diet and exercise plan outlined by their health care team. This plan is customized for each woman and is necessary for a healthy pregnancy outcome.

CAUSES OF GESTATIONAL DIABETES

Gestational diabetes is usually diagnosed or develops during pregnancy. It is characterized by hyperglycemia that is first observed during pregnancy. Glucose intolerance occurs during pregnancy and is synonymous with gestational diabetes.

The most common causes of gestational diabetes include a family history of diabetes, a previous 9-pound baby born to the same mother, overweight or loss, polycystic ovary syndrome (PCOS), African or Hispanic descent, obesity, recurrent infections and death. A newborn baby, or a mysterious miscarriage. Families in certain areas may be at higher risk. Women in South Asia, including India and Pakistan, are at risk.

Therefore, women in Middle Eastern countries such as Saudi Arabia, United Arab Emirates, Iraq, Jordan, Syria, Oman, Qatar, Kuwait, Lebanon and Egypt may also be susceptible to gestational diabetes. Women appear to have some degree of glucose intolerance due to hormonal changes during pregnancy. This means your blood sugar is higher than normal, but your diabetes is not. In the third trimester, the last trimester of pregnancy, these hormonal changes put women at risk for gestational diabetes. High levels of certain hormones made in the placenta transfer nutrients from the mother to the developing fetus. The placenta is the organ that connects the baby to the uterus through the umbilical cord.

However, residual hormones produced in the placenta help the mother prevent hypoglycemia from occurring, causing insulin to fail. As pregnancy progresses, these hormones eventually lead to impaired glucose tolerance, or high blood sugar. be connected. When blood sugar levels drop, the body produces more insulin, which rushes into cells to use for energy. The mother's pancreas may be able to produce three times as much insulin as she normally would. I have. This system produces blood sugar hormones to overcome the effects of pregnancy. When the pancreas cannot produce enough insulin to overcome the effects of increased hormones during pregnancy, blood sugar levels rise and gestational diabetes develops.

In addition, gestational diabetes or gestational diabetes mellitus (GDM) is a condition in which pregnant women present with hypertension without prior diagnosis of diabetes. Mothers with gestational diabetes give birth to babies with typical problems. These include birth complications, hypoglycemia, and jaundice. By controlling blood sugar levels, you can lower blood sugar levels. A woman with gestational diabetes is at increased risk of developing type 2 diabetes or potentially autoimmune type 1 diabetes after pregnancy. Children are said to be prone to childhood obesity, and type 2 diabetes develops later in life. Patients usually follow a moderate diet, exercise, or insulin.

CHAPTER FOUR

FOOD TO EAT OR AVOID (TYPE ONE DIABETES)

Choose healthful protein foods

Including protein in all meals helps balance blood sugar levels. People should choose healthy protein foods and vary their choices. Examples of these foods include:

- lean meat and poultry
- fish
- eggs
- beans and lentils
- tofu
- nuts and seeds
- low fat dairy foods

Eat plenty of Non-starchy vegetables

People should include plenty of non-starchy vegetables in their diet. According to the ADA, diets that consist primarily of plant-based foods, such as Mediterranean, vegan, and vegetarian diets, are beneficial for diabetes, weight loss, and blood pressure. Yes, non-starchy vegetables are high in fiber and have less of an impact on blood sugar than starchy vegetables. Non-starchy vegetables include:

- greens, such as lettuce, kale, cabbage, pak-choi, spinach, rocket, and watercress
- bell peppers
- zucchini and eggplant
- green beans
- mushrooms
- broccoli and cauliflower

Starchy vegetables like potatoes, pumpkin, and corn are high in sugar. However, people can include these in small amounts in their diets as long as they monitor their blood sugar levels.

Include nuts, seeds, beans, and legumes

Nuts, seeds, beans and legumes are good sources of fiber and can slow the release of sugars into the blood. They are also sources of protein. Examples of these foods are:

- Nuts: walnuts, Brazil nuts, almonds, and hazelnuts
- Seeds: chia, hemp, pumpkin, and sunflower seeds
- Beans and legumes: black beans, kidney beans, pintos, lentils, and garbanzo beans

Choose whole grains

You should choose whole grains instead of refined grains. Whole grains are a source of carbohydrates, but because they contain fiber, they have a better effect on blood sugar than refined grains. Recommended whole grains include:

- brown rice
- whole wheat bread
- whole grain pasta
- oatmeal
- other whole grains, such as buckwheat, quinoa, and millet

Opt for healthful fats

Including healthy fats in the diet can help someone feel fuller and avoid overeating carbohydrates. Healthy fats include:

- avocados

> olives and olive oil
> nuts and seeds
> oily fish, such as salmon, tuna, and mackerel

Stay hydrated

Staying hydrated is very important for people with type 1 diabetes because less water in the body means higher blood sugar levels. Water is the best way to stay hydrated, but you can also add citrus slices or mint to make flavored water or drink herbal tea.

Foods to avoid

Foods to avoid or limit include:

> added sugars
> refined grains, such as white bread, pasta, and rice
> processed foods
> sugary breakfast cereals
> sweet treats, such as cakes, biscuits, pastries, and candies
> soda, diet soda, and other sugary drinks
> juice drinks
> fried foods and food high in saturated and trans fats
> alcoholic beverages

CHAPTER FIVE

FOOD TO EAT OR AVOID (TYPE TWO DIABETES)

Vegetables

Vegetables form the basis of a nutritious diet. An excellent source of vitamins, minerals and fiber. The fiber and complex carbohydrates found in many vegetables help a person feel full. This helps prevent overeating, which can lead to unwanted weight gain and blood sugar problems. vegetable:

- broccoli
- carrots
- greens
- peppers
- tomatoes
- potatoes
- corn
- green peas

Beans and legumes

Beans, lentils, and other legumes are excellent sources of fiber and protein. The high fiber content of legumes means that the digestive tract absorbs fewer carbohydrates than low-fiber, high-carbohydrate foods. This makes these foods a good carbohydrate choice for diabetics. People can also use them in place of meat and cheese. Below are some examples of legumes that are available in canned, frozen, or dried form.

- black beans
- lentils
- white beans
- garbanzo beans

> kidney beans
> pinto beans

Pressure-cooked or slow-cooked beans also help improve digestibility.

Fruit

Fruits can be high in sugar, but the sugar content in whole fruit is not considered free sugar. Therefore, people with diabetes should not go without fruit. The following fruits are reliable additions to the diet of people with type 2 diabetes due to their low glycemic load.

> apples
> avocado
> blackberries
> cherries
> grapefruit
> peaches
> pears
> plums
> strawberries

Whole grains

Whole grains are an effective way to control blood sugar levels, as people with diabetes often have low blood sugar levels. People should avoid bleached and refined carbohydrates like white bread and white pasta and instead choose some of the options below when consuming grains:

> 100% whole wheat or legume-based pasta
> whole grain bread with at least 3 grams of fiber per slice
> quinoa
> wild rice

- ➢ 100% whole grain or whole wheat flour
- ➢ cornmeal
- ➢ oatmeal
- ➢ millet
- ➢ amaranth
- ➢ barley

Whole grains can also make you feel fuller for longer and add more flavor than highly processed carbohydrates.

Dairy

Dairy products contain essential nutrients such as calcium and protein. Some studies suggest that dairy products may have beneficial effects on insulin secretion in her type 2 diabetic patients. Some of the best options to add to your diet are:

- ➢ Parmesan, ricotta, or cottage cheese
- ➢ low fat or skim milk
- ➢ low fat Greek or plain yogurt

Meat

Protein is important for diabetics. Like high-fiber and high-fat foods, protein is slow to digest and only slightly raises blood sugar levels. Below are some good protein sources to choose from:

- ➢ skinless, boneless chicken breast or strips
- ➢ salmon, sardines, tuna, and other oily fish
- ➢ white fish fillets
- ➢ skinless turkey breast
- ➢ eggs

Plant-based proteins include beans and bean products, such as:

> ➢ black beans
> ➢ kidney beans
> ➢ pinto beans
> ➢ refried beans
> ➢ hummus
> ➢ falafel
> ➢ lentils
> ➢ peas
> ➢ edamame
> ➢ tempeh
> ➢ tofu

Dressings, dips, spices, and condiments

Many flavors and dressings are great for those trying to control their blood sugar levels. Below are some delicious options for diabetics to choose from:

> ➢ vinegar
> ➢ olive oil
> ➢ mustard
> ➢ any spice or herb
> ➢ any variety of extract
> ➢ hot sauce
> ➢ salsa

For a vinaigrette, whisk together equal parts olive oil and balsamic or other vinegar and season with salt, pepper, mustard, and herbs. Don't forget to consider the carbs your dressing provides. Barbecue sauce, ketchup, and certain salad dressings can also be high in fat, sugar, or both, so check your nutrition before buying these products. It is necessary to confirm the display.

Dessert foods

Desserts can be eaten by people with type 2 diabetes, but they should be careful about how much and how often they eat these foods. dessert options:

- ➢ popsicles with no added sugar
- ➢ 100% fruit popsicles
- ➢ sugar-free gelatin

Pudding or ice cream sweetened with zero or low-calorie sweeteners such as stevia or erythritol. Fruit-based desserts, such as homemade no-sugar fruit salads and summer fruit mixes, are a delicious and healthy way to end a meal. However, when counting carbs, it's wise to consider the sugar content in fruit.

Sugar-free options for diabetes

People with diabetes need to control their sugar intake. However, even sugar-free foods can affect blood sugar levels. "Sugar-free" means no sugar has been added to the food, but the product itself may contain carbohydrates that affect blood sugar levels. Sugar alcohols are an example. Manufacturers often use these low-calorie sweeteners in sugar-free chewing gum, candy, ice cream, and fruit spreads. Common sugar alcohols are:

- ➢ xylitol
- ➢ erythritol
- ➢ sorbitol
- ➢ maltitol

These are types of carbohydrates and can raise blood sugar levels. A person may want to opt for a sugar substitute, and in most cases his serving of the sugar substitute has little effect on blood sugar levels. Common sugar substitutes include:

- ➢ saccharin
- ➢ neotame
- ➢ aspartame
- ➢ sucralose
- ➢ stevia
- ➢ advantame

Snacks

For cravings between meals, a person can try:

- ➢ homemade popcorn, but not ready-made or sweetened varieties
- ➢ nuts, but not sweetened ones
- ➢ carrot or celery sticks with hummus
- ➢ small amounts of fresh fruit paired with a protein or fat, such as an apple with almond butter

Drinks

Water is healthy for everyone, including diabetics. There are other options, but drinks such as milk and juice are high in carbohydrates and can affect blood sugar levels. Here are some options that diabetics can consider:

- ➢ unsweetened ice or hot tea
- ➢ unsweetened coffee
- ➢ low fat or skim milk
- ➢ unsweetened plant-based milks
- ➢ sparkling water

FOODS TO LIMIT OR AVOID

People with type 2 diabetes should limit or avoid the same foods that are unhealthy for people without diabetes. You should also avoid foods that cause rapid fluctuations in blood sugar levels. People following a low-carb or low-carb diet plan should avoid consuming large amounts of:

➢ simple carbohydrates
➢ saturated and trans fats
➢ sugar in the form of candy, ice cream, and cakes

More specifically, people should limit their intake of:

➢ packaged and fast foods, such as baked goods, sweets, chips, and desserts
➢ white bread
➢ white pasta
➢ white rice
➢ fried foods such as French fries
➢ sugary cereals
➢ sugary drinks
➢ processed meats
➢ red meat

We also recommend avoiding low-fat products that replace fat with sugar. Fat-free yogurt is a good example. People with prediabetes or type 2 diabetes can try replacing some foods with healthier versions. This includes choosing brown rice, pasta, or bread, or substituting baked potatoes for baked potatoes. Cooking food at home is usually the best option because it allows people to avoid the added sugar found in many prepared foods.

Understanding food packaging

Food packaging can be confusing. Most foods need labels with nutritional information, but many people don't read them or know what to look for. Below are some tips to help you better understand the packaging labels and messages:

Read the nutrition facts label: Just because a food claims to be low in fat or sugar doesn't mean it really is. Find and read the nutrition information label on the package to understand what the food contains. is important.

Look for specific nutrition facts: Information can confuse many people. The most important information for diabetics to look out for is the total grams of carbohydrates per serving and serving size.

Count carbohydrates: Fiber is a type of carbohydrate and may appear under the total carbohydrates list. The body does not digest fiber, so a person can subtract it from the total carbohydrates in the diet. A more accurate way to count.

Read the ingredients list: The ingredient list is ordered from highest to lowest total content. If sugar is on top, it's the main ingredient.

Look for hidden sources of sugar: Sugar appears under many different names on ingredient lists, including corn syrup, fructose, and dextrose. Recognizing sugar's multiple identities can help shoppers avoid adding sugar of any kind.

Limit or avoid artificial sweeteners: Older research from credible sources suggests that artificial sweeteners may have adverse health effects and promote sweet cravings. But not all scientists agree. Popular artificial sweeteners include aspartame, sucralose, neotame, saccharin and acesulfame potassium.

Sample grocery list

Grocery lists typically change from week to week based on a person's needs and desires. However, consider using the following sample list as a starting point.

- apples
- tomatoes
- whole strawberries
- fresh or frozen vegetables or both
- corn
- cucumber
- fresh basil
- a bagged salad
- onion
- red bell pepper
- romaine lettuce
- yellow or green squash or zucchini
- boneless, skinless chicken breasts
- wild-caught salmon fillet
- unsweetened almond or flax milk
- 1–2% milk
- fresh mozzarella cheese
- Parmesan cheese
- sweet potatoes
- wild rice mix
- honey
- unsweetened, olive oil-based dressing
- low sugar, low sodium barbecue sauce
- olive oil
- olive oil spray
- black pepper
- reduced sodium soy sauce
- salt
- coffee
- walnuts, almonds, or other raw nuts

CHAPTER SIX

FOOD TO EAT OR AVOID (GESTATIONAL DIABETES)

What foods should I eat?

This is one of the most common questions pregnant women ask when being diagnosed with gestational diabetes. It can feel like you can't eat, especially if you're new to insulin or have severe insulin resistance.

Some foods you should eat are:

- Plenty of green, leafy vegetables, like kale, spinach, cabbage, and romaine lettuce
- Bright vegetables, like bell peppers, carrots, sweet potatoes, and squashes
- Lots of fresh fruit, including strawberries, blueberries, raspberries, and coconut
- Whole grains, like steel-cut oatmeal, whole-grain breads, and pastas
- Healthy fats, like avocados, extra virgin olive oil, seeds, and nuts
- Lean proteins, like chicken and turkey, eggs and egg whites
- Fish, like salmon, mackerel, and white fish
- Healthy dairy, like lower-fat cheese, Greek yogurt, kefir, and low-fat milk

Eat 3 meals and 2–3 snacks per day

Eating too much at once (especially too many carbs) can cause blood sugar to rise too high, so eating small meals and snacks can help blood sugar control.

Choose healthier carbohydrates

The types of carbohydrates you eat and drink have a big impact on your blood sugar levels. Choosing carbs that are minimally processed, low in simple sugars, and have a low glycemic index can help keep blood sugar levels stable. It includes complex carbohydrates such as non-starchy vegetables, oats, brown rice and whole grain bread.

Eat plenty of fiber

Dietary fiber slows digestion and helps extract nutrients from what you eat better. Since high-fiber foods are digested more slowly, they also help reduce blood sugar spikes after meals.

Good sources of fiber are:

- Beans and peas
- Low-carb fruits
- Oats (such as oat bran and oatmeal)
- Nuts and seeds
- Vegetables (such as cauliflower and green beans)
- Wheat bran
- Whole-grain foods (such as brown rice and whole-grain bread, cereals, and pasta)

Include protein in every meal

Protein is a building block of muscles and ligaments and is essential for muscle growth. Getting enough protein is important for both you and your baby. Also, protein does not raise blood sugar levels. Normally, pregnant women are recommended to consume 6-8 ounces of protein per day, but work with your doctor to find the right amount for you.

Good sources of protein are:

> - Lean beef or veal
> - Cheese
> - Chicken
> - Cottage cheese
> - Egg
> - Fish and seafood (but read below about what fish and seafood to avoid)
> - Pork
> - Turkey
> - Tofu
> - Edamame
> - Nuts/seeds

What foods should I avoid?

What you avoid may be more important than what you eat. The following foods can increase inflammation, worsen blood sugar levels, increase insulin resistance, and make gestational diabetes more difficult to manage:

> - Sugar-sweetened beverages, like juice, sweet tea, and soda
> - Energy drinks with excess caffeine
> - High-calorie, high-sodium fast food (burgers, fries, etc.)
> - Fried foods, like French fries and chips
> - Highly processed foods
> - Food with added sugar, like ice cream, cakes, donuts, muffins, and cookies
> - High-fat red meats (lean cuts are fine)
> - Alcoholic beverages
> - Candy, like taffy and chocolates
> - Refined grains, including white pasta and white rice
> - Boxed cereals and sugar-sweetened granola bars and granola with more than 10 grams of sugar per serving
> - Sweetened yogurts and milk products

Be careful with fish and shellfish

Seafood is healthy and should be included in a diet for gestational diabetes, but some species should be limited or avoided. Large predatory fish such as swordfish, sharks and marlin can be harmful to you and your baby. can accumulate significant mercury and other toxins and should be avoided altogether. Oily fish such as salmon, trout, mackerel and herring should be consumed in excess of 2 servings (8-12 ounces) per week. Please don't eat it. Fatty fish may contain more contaminants than other types of fish. Tuna (raw or canned) should also be limited to two servings per week, as tuna is also high in mercury. Avoid raw shellfish altogether, as they can contain harmful bacteria, viruses, or toxins that can lead to food poisoning.

Avoid raw or undercooked meats

Eating raw or undercooked meat poses a small risk of contracting toxoplasmosis and may lead to miscarriage. As well as raw meat, salami, pepperoni, and chorizo, which may not be fully cooked Smoked meats such as prosciutto and cold cuts should also be avoided. Liver products such as liver and pies also contain high levels of vitamin A which can be harmful to babies and should be avoided.

Avoid unpasteurized milk and cheese

Pasteurization is the heating of milk or dairy products to 72°C for 15 seconds to kill pathogens harmful to humans. Unpasteurized dairy products have a lower risk of containing listeria monocytogenes, which can cause listeriosis and lead to miscarriage and stillbirth. It is also recommended to avoid cooked cheese. This is because the coating can promote bacterial growth.

CHAPTER SEVEN

MEAL PLAN FOR TYPE ONE DIABETES

Creating a type 1 diabetes meal plan

People can use a variety of methods to plan their diet for type 1 diabetes. You can also ask a nutritionist for help. Common meal preparation methods include:

Carbohydrate counting: This method tracks how many grams of carbs you eat or drink each day.

Glycemic index: Glycemic index (GI) and glycemic load (GL) measure the amount of sugars in foods and how much they raise blood sugar levels.

Plate method: People can use this technology to control portion sizes and food groups. Half of the plate consists of non-starchy vegetables, one quarter contains healthy protein, and the last quarter contains Filled with grains or starch.

Type 1 diabetes snacks

Snacks should aim to balance carbs with protein or fat. There are also so-called diabetic sweets, which should be kept to a minimum. Here are some healthy snack ideas:

➢ chocolate protein balls made with oats, nut butter, cocoa powder, and a diabetes-friendly sweetener, such as stevia
➢ celery sticks and nut butter
➢ a boiled egg
➢ hummus and oatcakes

People who keep track of their carbohydrate intake should count whenever they eat fruit as a snack. A small piece of whole fruit contains about 15g of carbohydrates. Berries are a lower GI fruit, and melons, pineapples, and some dried fruits have a medium GI.

Eating low-sugar fruit along with a protein source may help balance blood sugar better than eating fruit alone. For example, someone might be eating berries with plain yogurt.

CHAPTER EIGHT

MEAL PLAN FOR TYPE TWO DIABETES

DAY 1

You can control your blood sugar levels by eating a diabetic-friendly diet. But sticking to a regular eating plan can be difficult unless you have a plan.

Check out those 21 delicious, diabetes-pleasant recipes to apply for breakfast, lunch, and dinner. Remember to stay within your carbohydrate intake by paying attention to the carbohydrate content and serving sizes in your recipes. Also, balance your diet with lean protein and healthier vegetable fats.

Breakfast: Cream Cheese-Stuffed French Toast

It may sound greasy for breakfast, but when paired with scrambled eggs, it fits into a diabetes-friendly meal plan. Whole grain toast can help ensure you're getting your daily fiber as well.

Lunch: Salmon Salad with White Beans

One of the best sources of omega-3 fatty acids, salmon is a delicious topping for your everyday salad.

Dinner: Cuban-Marinated Sirloin Kabobs with Grilled Asparagus

Spice it up with these appetizing skewers. Dried herbs and spices are a great way to pack in flavor without adding unnecessary calories and fat.

DAY 2

Breakfast: Apple Pie Oatmeal with Greek Yogurt

Who doesn't want cake for breakfast? This oatmeal will make your kitchen smell like the tastes of autumn and leave your stomach happy and satisfied. Add plain Greek yogurt on top for more protein.

Lunch: Turkey-Cranberry Wraps

Turkey and cranberry sauce are not only for Thanksgiving! This is a smooth grab-and-move lunch that even your children will enjoy.

Note: This recipe has 34 grams of carbohydrates per serving, so it may not be suitable for everyone with type 2 diabetes. You can adjust the amount of cranberry sauce to reduce the number of carbohydrates.

Dinner: Cilantro-Lime Tilapia with Spinach and Tomatoes

Take a trip to the tropics with this easy seafood dish.

DAY 3

Breakfast: Fruit and Almond Smoothie

If you think you're too busy to eat breakfast in the morning, think again. This smoothie consists of just four ingredients and is ready in no time.

Lunch: Veggie and Chicken Pasta Salad

This pasta dish is perfect for dinner as well as lunch. Make two batches later in the week for leftovers.

Dinner: Grilled Turkey Burgers

Burgers are really healthy and delicious. Top off your meal with oven-baked sweet potato fries for a drive-thru meal at home.

DAY 4

Breakfast: Veggie and Goat Cheese Scramble

When your taste buds are craving delectable stuffs in the morning, these veggie and egg scrambled eggs are for you. Sautéed peppers and tomatoes combine with eggs, avocado and cheese for a mouthwatering and hearty meal. breakfast plate.

Lunch: Curried Chicken Salad Stuffed Pitas

This chicken sandwich features creamy Greek yogurt mayonnaise.

Dinner: Jamaican Pork Tenderloin with Lemony Green Beans

This quick and easy dinner is enough for a summer treat. Enjoy with brown rice or pilaf.

DAY 5

Breakfast: Granola with Nuts, Seeds, and Dried Fruit

Make this granola over the weekend and divide it into a week's worth of breakfasts for you and your family.

Note: This recipe is high in sugar because it contains dried fruit. You can adjust it by removing the dried fruit.

Lunch: Quinoa Tabbouleh Salad

Quinoa is naturally gluten-free and, as one of the few plant-based foods, is also considered a complete protein. Vegetarians and carnivores alike will enjoy this Arabian salad.

Dinner: Beef and Rice Stuffed Peppers

Stuffed peppers are a sophisticated, family-friendly option that's perfect for any night of the week.

DAY 6

Breakfast: Banana-Carrot and Pecan Muffins

Serve these muffins at your next brunch and everyone will almost certainly be begging for the recipe!

Lunch: Lemony Hummus

hummus gotten from store can be salty and tasteless. By making your own, you can reduce the salt content and adjust the seasoning to your liking. Hummus can be paired with vegetables (carrots, radishes, celery, sliced cucumbers, green peppers) and foods such as pita chips, bread and whole grain crackers.

Dinner: Chicken Tortilla Soup

Do you have leftover cooked chicken? Enjoy the umami-filled soup that will definitely fill you up!

DAY 7

Breakfast: Tomato and Basil Frittata

Frittatas are a considerable means to use up surplus ingredients. Serve with whole grain toast and sliced fruit for a full weekend breakfast.

Lunch: Butternut Squash and Carrot Soup

Once you try this soup, chances are you won't be able to go back to the canned variety.

Dinner: Grilled Shrimp Skewers

Shrimp takes only a few minutes to cook. So, when it hits the grill, it's dinner time.

CHAPTER NINE

MEAL PLAN FOR GESTATIONAL DIABETES

3-Day Gestational Diabetes Meal Plan

This simple gestational diabetes meal plan shows what a healthy eating day looks like. You can follow this plan as-is or use it as a template to create your own healthy gestational diabetes meal plan. Please create a meal plan.

DAY 1

Breakfast: Old-Fashioned Oatmeal

AM Snack: 1/3 cup raw almonds + ½ cup mixed berries

Lunch: Salmon Salad

PM Snack: Lime & Parmesan Popcorn

Dinner: Zucchini Noodles with Quick Turkey Bolognese

DAY 2

Breakfast: Florentine Hash Skillet

AM Snack: 1 small apple + 2 Tbsp. almond butter

Lunch: Cherry, Wild Rice & Quinoa Salad

PM Snack: 1 cup vegetable of choice + ½ cup hummus

Dinner: Very Green Lentil Soup

DAY 3

Breakfast: ½ cup plain Greek yogurt + ½ cup blueberries + 1 Tbsp. chia seeds

AM Snack: Frozen Chocolate-Banana Bites

Lunch: Veggie & Hummus Sandwich

PM Snack: Guacamole-Stuffed Egg

Dinner: Roast Chicken with Parmesan-Herb Sauce

CHAPTER TEN

RECIPES FOR TYPE ONE DIABETES

Breakfast: Oatmeal pecan pancakes

A healthy start to the day, these pancakes are loaded with whole grain oats and delicious pecans.

Ingredients (6 servings):

Oats	1 cup
Baking powder	1 1/2 tsp
Eggs	2
Skimmed milk	1/3 cup
Mashed banana	1/3 cup
Vanilla extract	1/2 tsp
Chopped pecans	2 tbsp
Canola oil	1 tbsp

Method:

Place the oatmeal and baking soda in a food processor and set aside. Mix eggs, milk, vanilla extract and mashed bananas, add oatmeal and pecans. Pour 1/4 cup of mixture into oiled skillet and sear on both sides.

Lunch: Power lunch salad

A nutritious salad with a good balance of vegetables, protein and carbohydrates.

Ingredients (4 servings):

Baby spinach	5 1/2 oz
Almonds (sliced)	2 tbsp
Pepitas (dry roasted)	1/4 cup
Dried cranberries	1/2 cup
Small apple (diced)	1
Reduced fat feta cheese	1/3 cup
Oven roasted deli turkey breast	7 oz
Balsamic vinegar	1/3 cup
Olive oil	1 1/2 tbsp

Method:

Mix entire salad ingredients in a salad bowl. Make a dressing by mixing the vinegar and oil and drizzle it over the salad.

Dinner: Alaska salmon with orange and watercress

A delicious and nutritious dinner packed with healthy fats.

Ingredients (8 servings):

Alaska salmon fillets (4–6 oz each)	4
Avocado oil	1/4 cup
Watercress (roughly chopped)	3 cups
Cucumber (finely chopped)	3 tbsp
Orange (peeled and separated into segments)	2

White wine vinegar	1 tsp
Salt and pepper	1 pinch
Mixed greens	2 cups
Avocado (sliced)	½
Walnuts	1/4 cup
Apple cider vinegar	2 tbsp
Pimentos (smoked paprika — optional topping)	1 pinch
Nasturtiums (edible flowers — optional topping)	4

Method:

Step 1: Brush both sides of salmon with avocado oil and sear in skillet over medium-high heat, 4 minutes per side until browned. Flip the salmon over and season the other side with salt and pepper. Cook salmon until opaque throughout.

Step 2: Place the watercress, cucumber, and orange pieces in a bowl and season with white wine vinegar, avocado oil, and salt and pepper.

Step 3: Serve all and top with avocado, walnuts, apple cider vinegar and optional nasturtium.

Preparing meals for children with diabetes

When preparing meals for children with diabetes, the same healthy eating principles apply as for adults. For example, it's important to avoid processed foods and packaged breakfast cereals because they're high in sugar. Preparing packed lunches for kids makes it easier to monitor food groups and portions.

Healthy back-to-school lunch

It's easy to make, and it's a healthy and delicious bento that's perfect for lunch.

Ingredients (1 serving):

Hummus	1 tsp
Cucumber	4 slices
Greek yogurt tube (2 oz)	1 packet
Blueberries and sliced strawberries	1/2 cup
Cheddar cheese (reduced fat)	1/2 oz
Sunflower seeds	1 tsp
Mustard	1 tsp
Romaine lettuce leaf	1
Whole grain dinner roll	1
Deli-style turkey breast (no added salt)	2 oz

Method:

Spread mustard on the roll and put turkey, cheese and lettuce in between to make a sandwich. For a snack, spread hummus on cucumber slices and top with sunflower seeds. Put it all in your lunch box.

CHAPTER ELEVEN

RECIPES FOR TYPE TWO DIABETES

Cream Cheese-Stuffed French Toast

Ingredients

½ cup	Fat-free cream cheese (about 5 ounces)
2 tbs	Strawberry or apricot spreadable fruit
8 1-inch Slice	French bread
2	Egg whites
1	Egg, slightly beaten
¾ cup	Fat-free milk
½ tbs	Vanilla
1/8 tbs	Apple pie spice
	Nonstick cooking spray
½ cup	Strawberry or apricot spreadable fruit

Directions

Step 1: In a small bowl, combine cream cheese and 2 tablespoons spread fruit. Using a serrated knife, make a pocket in each slice of bread and cut horizontally halfway between the top and bottom crust, rather than cutting all the way through. Add a tablespoon of cream cheese mixture to each pocket. Add about 1 scoop (see Tips).

Step 2: In a small bowl, mix egg whites, eggs, milk, vanilla and apple pie spice. Lightly coat a nonstick griddle with cooking spray. Heat over medium heat.

Step 3: Dip the stuffed bread slices into the egg mixture and brush on both sides. Place bread slices on hot griddle. Cook, flipping once, about 3 minutes or until golden brown.

Step 4: Meanwhile, in a small saucepan, heat 1/2 cup spread fruit, stirring frequently, until melted. Spread over French toast.

Tips

To make ahead: Stuff each slice of bread and place in an airtight container. Cover; refrigerate overnight. Prepare and cook the egg mixture in the morning.

Salmon Salad with White Beans

Ingredients (Makes 4 servings)

½ pound	Salmon steak (leftover grilled salmon is fine)
1/3 cup	Extra-virgin olive oil,
½ tbs	Dried thyme, if using raw fish
1	Red or yellow bell pepper
	Juice of 1 large lemon, plus more to taste if necessary
2 cups	Cooked or canned white beans, drained
10	Cherry tomatoes, halved
¼ cup	Diced shallots
12 to 15	Good black or green olives, pitted and coarsely chopped
¼ cup	Minced fresh basil leaves
¼ cup	Minced fresh parsley leaves
	Salt and freshly ground black pepper to taste
	Freshly ground black pepper

| 4 cups | Torn assorted salad greens (trimmed, washed and dried) |

Directions

Step 1: If starting with raw salmon, start a charcoal or wood fire, or preheat a gas or grill. The rack should be approximately 4 inches away from the heat source. Marinate fish in 2 tablespoons olive oil and thyme.

Step 2: Once done (it should be fairly hot), sear the fish for 3-4 minutes on each side. Roast red peppers at the same time. Cool, peel, core and cut into strips.

Step 3: Chill the fish, cut it into small cubes, toss with the lemon juice, beans and remaining olive oil and prepare the other ingredients. Add tomatoes, shallots, olives, and herbs to salmon. Season with salt and pepper and adjust the balance of olive oil and lemon juice if necessary. Serve over leafy greens and garnish with grilled red pepper.

Cuban-Marinated Sirloin Kabobs with Grilled Asparagus

This Latin-inspired steak goes great with rice or beans. The diced leftovers are very thin and can be served with his crispy day-old buns after a great lunch or snack. This is one of his kind recipes to add to your routine. Whenever you're looking for something different to eat, this should be on your list. The Cuban Marinated Roast Beef Kebab with Grilled Asparagus is a must try.

Marinated Roast Beef Kebab with Grilled Asparagus is a very simple and easy recipe. It's also a great accompaniment to a main course. You can enjoy it as is.

For grilled asparagus-

Ingredients

1-pound	Fresh asparagus
1 tbs	Extra virgin olive oil
¼ tbs	Kosher salt
½ tbs	Fresh pepper

Directions

Step 1: Remove thin ends of asparagus. To do this, hold the spear and gently bend it until it is naturally soft. This removes the lower third of the spear.

Step 2: Arrange the asparagus on a flat plate. Sprinkle with olive oil, sprinkle with salt and pepper, and coat all over.

Step 3: Arrange asparagus in grill pan or evenly perforated aluminum foil. Sauté over medium heat for 5 minutes or until browned on all sides.

For the kabobs:

Ingredients

400g	Chives
½ cup	Finely chopped onion
½ cup	Orange juice
¼ cup	Lime juice
2 tbs	Chopped fresh garlic
1 tbs	Dried oregano
1 tbs	Baked cumin
1 tbs	Extra virgin olive oil

½ tbs	Kosher salt
½ tbs	Fresh pepper
	Glue wedges (optional)

Directions

Step 1: Trim excess fat and cut into 1-inch cubes. Place the meat in a tight plastic bag.

Step 2: Stir in the onion, orange and lime juice, garlic, oregano, and cumin. Pour over the meat. Dry the bag and shake it gently to evenly coat the meat with the marinade.

Step 3: Chill for at least 4 hours.

Step 4: After marinating, dry the meat with paper towels. Rub meat evenly with olive oil, then season with salt and pepper.

Step 5: Thread the meat onto wooden skewers. Grill over medium heat for 8-10 minutes or until desired thickness, flipping every 2 minutes to sear on both sides.

Step 6: Served with grilled asparagus and lime wedges.

Notes-

For maximum flavor, marinate the fillet for at least 4 hours, preferably overnight. Before grilling the meat, soak the wooden skewers in warm water for an hour to prevent the meat from burning. Complete your meal with a choice of steamed brown rice, orzo, or whole grain couscous.

Apple Pie Oatmeal with Greek Yogurt

Ingredients

1/3 cup	Quick oats
2/3 cup	Milk
¼ cup	Greek vanilla yogurt
¼ cup	Apple sauce
¼ cup	Chopped fresh apple
1 tbs	Raisins
	Dash cinnamon
	Sprinkle shredded coconut

Directions

Step 1: Mix oatmeal and milk and bring to a boil. I cook in the microwave, but you can cook on the stove as well.

Step 2: Putting it all together:

- Add 1/4 cup vanilla Greek yogurt to the cooked oatmeal.
- Add applesauce, chopped apples, and raisins.
- Sprinkle with cinnamon and coconut flakes.
- Enjoy!

Turkey-Cranberry Wraps

Ingredients

2 ½ tbs	Whipped reduced-fat cream cheese spread
1	Light Original Flatbread
1 cup	Torn romaine lettuce
3-ounces	Sliced cooked turkey or chicken breast meat
2 tbs	Reduced-sugar or light cranberry sauce

Directions

Step 1: Spread cream cheese on one side of the flatbread. Topped with romaine, turkey and cranberry sauce. Roll the flatbread around the filling.

Cilantro-Lime Tilapia with Spinach and Tomatoes

Ingredients

1(4-ounce)	Tilapia fillet
1 tbs	Olive oil
	Juice from half a lime
	Garlic/garlic powder (optional)
½ tbs	Chopped fresh cilantro
½ cup	Cooked spinach
¼ cup	Chopped fresh tomatoes

Tips:

We love this dinner served with asparagus.

Directions

Step 1: Preheat the grill.

Step 2: Brush the tilapia with olive oil.

Step 3: Squeeze lime juice, then sprinkle with garlic powder and coriander (optional).

Step 4: Bake in the oven over 6 inches of heat for about 5 to 7 minutes or until the fish flakes easily with a fork.

Step 5: While the tilapia is cooking, place the spinach in a microwave-safe bowl.

Step 6: Stir in garlic powder or minced garlic (optional).

Step 7: Prepare according to package directions.

Step 8: Cover and keep warm until filet is done.

Step 9: Place the cooked spinach on a plate, place the fish on the spinach and top with the chopped tomatoes.

Step 10: Serve with herb bread if desired.

The recipe is for one person. Multiply by the number of servings the recipe calls for. (As a dinner for 1-12 people!)

Fruit and Almond Smoothie

Ingredients

Frozen strawberries and peaches	1 cup
Plain Nonfat Greek yogurt	1/2 cup
Unsweetened almond milk	1 cup

Directions

Step 1: Place all ingredients in a blender and blend until smooth and thick.

Veggie and Chicken Pasta Salad

Ingredients

Uncooked whole-wheat elbow pasta	1 cup
Diced red bell pepper	1/2 cup
Diced cucumber	1/2 cup
Small broccoli florets (fresh or frozen)	1/2 cup
Large carrot (diced)	1
Diced cooked chicken breast	1 cup
Light mayonnaise	1/4 cup
Red wine vinegar	1 tbsp
Dried oregano	1/8 tsp
Freshly ground black pepper	1/8 tsp

Directions

Step 1: Prepare the pasta according to the package directions. Drain.

Step 2: In a large bowl, combine pasta, red peppers, cucumbers, broccoli, carrots and chicken.

Step 3: Combine the dressing ingredients in a small bowl and mix. Pour the dressing over the pasta, vegetables, and chicken and mix well. additional fee.

Grilled Turkey Burgers

Ingredients

1-pound	93%-lean ground turkey
1	Small onion, grated
2 tbs	Ketchup
1 tbs	Worcestershire sauce
1 tbs	Dry mustard
¼ tbs	Salt
¼ tbs	Ground pepper
½ cup	Fresh whole-wheat breadcrumbs
4	Whole-wheat hamburger buns, toasted
	Lettuce, sliced red onion & tomato for serving

Directions

Step 1: In a medium bowl, combine turkey meat, grated onion, ketchup, Worcestershire sauce, dry mustard, salt, and pepper. Add bread crumbs and mix by hand until combined. Divide the mixture into four 1/2-inch thick he burgers. Cover and freeze for at least 15 minutes or up to 8 hours.

Step 2: Meanwhile, preheat grill to medium-high.

Step 3: Grease the grill grates. Grill burgers until instant-read thermometer reads 165°F in center, about 4 minutes per side. Place on a clean plate and let rest for 5 minutes. Serve on buns with lettuce, red onion and tomato, if desired.

To make ahead: Refrigerate burgers (Step 1) for up to 8 hours.

Veggie and Goat Cheese Scramble

Ingredients

1 tbs	Unsalted butter
8	Eggs, beaten
¾ cup	Milk
4-ounce	Goat cheese, crumbled
1 cup	Bell pepper, diced
½ cup	Halved cherry tomatoes
1	Avocado, diced
	Parsley, fresh ground black pepper to garnish

Directions

Step 1: Melt the butter in a large skillet over medium heat. Add the peppers, season with a little salt and pepper, and simmer for 4-5 minutes, until tender.

Step 2: While the peppers are cooking, whisk together the eggs, milk, cherry tomatoes, and 3/4 of the goat cheese.

Step 3: Lower the heat to medium and pour the egg mixture into the frying pan. Cook for 1-2 minutes until the eggs begin to set. Once the egg begins to set, gently pull the egg from the edge of the pan toward the center and fold it in, repeating the process until the egg sets (it should look a little shiny or wet on top, but not runny.).

Step 4: Top with avocado, leftover goat cheese crumble, parsley and pepper.

Curried Chicken Salad Stuffed Pitas

Ingredients

3 tbs	Hy-Vee mayonnaise
¼ cup	Hy-Vee plain Greek yogurt
1 tbs	Curry powder
	Hy-Vee salt, to taste
3 cups	Cooked chicken breast, or rotisserie chicken, shredded
1	Medium stalk celery, finely chopped
2	Green onions, chopped
1 cup	Red seedless grapes, halved
1 tbs	Fresh parsley, chopped
3	Whole wheat pita breads, halved

Things to grab

> ➢ Whisk
> ➢ Large bowl

Directions

Step 1: Combine mayonnaise, yogurt, curry powder and salt in a large bowl and mix well. Add chicken, celery, onions, grapes, and parsley.

Step 2: Add 1/2 cup chicken salad to each half of flatbread.

Jamaican Pork Tenderloin with Lemony Green Beans

Jamaican Pork Tenderloin:

Ingredients

2 tbs	Brown sugar
1 tbs	Ground allspice
1 tbs	Ground cinnamon
½ tbs	Ground ginger
½ tbs	Onion powder
½ tbs	Garlic powder
¼ tbs	Cayenne pepper
1/8 tbs	Ground cloves
¾ tbs	Salt
½ tbs	Ground black pepper freshly ground
1	Tenderloin about 1 pound, trimmed of visible fat
2 tbs	White vinegar
1 ½ tbs	Honey
1 tbs	Tomato paste

Directions

Step 1: In a small bowl mix the following: brown sugar, cinnamon, ginger, onion powder, allspice, garlic powder, cayenne, cloves, 1/2 teaspoon salt and black pepper. Rub spice mixture onto pork and let stand for 15 minutes.

Step 2: In another small bowl, mix vinegar, honey, tomato paste, and remaining 1/4 teaspoon salt. Mix with a whisk. set aside.

Step 3: Heat grill or broiler to medium-high or 400 F. Away from heat sources, lightly coat a grill grate or grill pan with cooking spray. Hold the cooking grate 4 to 6 inches away from the heat source.

Step 6: Place pork on grill grate or grill pan. Cook over medium-high heat, flipping several times, until browned on all sides, 3 to 4 minutes total. Place on a cool part of the grill or reduce the heat and cook for an additional 14 to 16 minutes. Dip the pork in the honey vinegar sauce until the pork is slightly pink inside and use an instant-read thermometer inserted in the thickest part. Continue cooking 3 to 4 minutes longer, until D reads 160 F. Place on cutting board and let cool 5 minutes before slicing.

Lemony Green Beans:

Ingredients

1-pound	Thin green beans
2 tbs	Butter
	Freshly squeezed lemon juice, to taste
¼ tbs	Salt
¼ tbs	Freshly ground black pepper

Directions

Step 1: Break the green bean stems or cut them off with a knife into large clusters.

Step 2: Heat a frying pan over medium heat and add butter. (Using a pan with a thin bottom helps keep an eye on the color.) Rotate the pan occasionally to help the butter cook evenly. As the butter melts it will start to bubble. The color goes from lemon yellow to golden yellow and finally to roast brown.

Step 3: When it smells fragrant, add green beans and fry for 3 to 4 minutes. Add some lemon juice, salt and pepper and use tongs to serve on a plate.

Granola with Nuts, Seeds, and Dried Fruit

Ingredients

8 cups	Rolled oats (not the quick kind)
1 cup	Sunflower seeds
½ cup	Pepitas
1 cup	Pecans roughly chopped
½ cup	Flaked almonds
1 cup	Walnuts roughly chopped
1 cup	Unsalted cashews (I left mine whole)
½ cup	Coconut flakes (or any kind of coconut that you like)
½ cup	Dried cranberries
½ cup	Sultanas (or raisins)
½ cup	Dried apricots, chopped
2 tbs	Vanilla extract (the good stuff)
1 cup	Oil (I used macadamia nut oil but anything will work)
¾ cup	Honey
¼ cup	Maple syrup
1 ½ tbs	Salt
½ cup	Brown sugar

Directions

Step 1: Preheat oven to 165°C.

Step 2: In the largest bowl, combine the oats, sunflower seeds, pepitas, pecans, almonds, coconut, walnuts and cashews and set aside.

Step 3: Bring maple syrup, honey, oil, sugar, vanilla and brown sugar to a boil in a large pot. After cooking for 5 minutes, the mixture will thicken slightly.

Step 4: Pour the hot mixture over the oatmeal, seeds and nuts and stir to coat.

Step 5: Place on a foil or parchment paper (I use foil) lined baking sheet and bake for 20 minutes. Halfway through baking, stir the granola to ensure all the granola is toasted.

Step 6: When the granola is light brown, remove it from the oven and stir in the sultanas, cranberries and apricots (or other dried fruit).

Step 7: Once completely cooled, store the granola in an airtight container for up to 2 weeks. (Mine hasn't been there for over a week)

Quinoa Tabbouleh Salad

Ingredients (Makes 6 servings)

1 cup	Quinoa, rinsed well
½ tbs	Kosher salt plus more
2 tbs	Fresh lemon juice
1	Garlic clove, minced
½ cup	Extra-virgin olive oil
	Freshly ground black pepper

1	Large English hothouse cucumber or 2 Persian cucumbers, cut into 1/4" pieces
1-pint	Cherry tomatoes, halved
2/3 cup	Chopped flat-leaf parsley
½ cup	Chopped fresh mint
2	Scallions, thinly sliced

Directions

Step 1: In a medium saucepan over high heat, bring quinoa, 1/2 teaspoon salt, and 1 1/4 cups water to a boil. Reduce heat to medium-low, cover, and simmer until quinoa is tender, about 10 minutes. Remove from stove and leave covered for 5 minutes. fluff with a fork.

Step 2: Meanwhile, whisk together the lemon juice and garlic in a small bowl. Add the olive oil little by little. Season the dressing with salt and pepper to taste.

Step 3: Spread quinoa on a large rimmed baking sheet. Let cool. Pour into a large bowl. Stir in 1/4 cup dressing. Get ahead: Available from 1 day in advance. Cover remaining dressing and quinoa separately. nice.

Step 4: Place the cucumbers, tomatoes, herbs, and green onions into the bowl with the quinoa. Toss for coating. Season with salt and pepper. Drizzle the rest of the dressing.

Beef and Rice Stuffed Peppers

Ingredients

6	Bell peppers
3 cups	Chunky tomato sauce, divided
½	Onion, very thinly sliced
1 cup	Beef broth
¼ tbs	Red pepper flakes
1 ½ pounds	Lean ground beef
1 ½ cups	Cooked rice
½ cup	Freshly shredded Parmigiano-Reggiano cheese
¼ cup	Chopped fresh flat-leaf parsley
4	Cloves garlic, minced
2 tbs	Salt
½ tbs	Freshly ground black pepper
1 tbs	Chopped fresh flat-leaf parsley, divided

Directions

Step 1: Preheat the oven to 190°C.

Step 2: Slice the peppers 1/2 inch from the top. Cut off the stem and set the tip aside. Cut the core out of the peppers and remove the seeds. Slice the pepper thinly from the bottom so that it is upright. Poke four small holes in the bottom to allow juices to drain.

Step 3: Pour 2 1/2 cups tomato sauce into a 9x13-inch casserole dish. Add onion, beef broth, and red pepper flakes. Spread out mixture evenly over the bottom. Place the peppers vertically on the plate.

Step 4: In a large mixing bowl, combine ground beef, cooked rice, Parmigiano-Reggiano cheese, 2 tablespoons tomato sauce, 1/4 cup parsley, garlic, salt, and black pepper.

Step 5: Lightly stuff peppers with meat mixture. Spread 1 tablespoon tomato sauce over each serving of filling. Place the reserved tops over the peppers. Place parchment paper loosely over peppers and cover plate tightly with foil. Place the mold on the baking sheet.

Step 6: Bake in preheated oven until peppers are tender, about 1 hour. Remove foil and parchment. Continue to bake for an additional 20-30 minutes until the meat filling is fully cooked and the peppers are tender.

Step 7: Sprinkle each pepper with 1/2 teaspoon of parsley and drizzle with 1 tablespoon of pan juices.

Chef's Notes:

I use parchment paper for this recipe because I don't like the foil touching anything acidic while baking. If you don't use the baking sheet, your peppers will bake faster.

Banana-Carrot and Pecan Muffins

Ingredients

1 cup	Whole wheat flour
1 tbs	Baking powder
1 tbs	Ground cinnamon
¼ tbs	Baking soda
½ tbs	Kosher salt
¼ cup	Canola oil
1/3 cup	Brown sugar
1	Large egg
1/3 cup	Vanilla sugar-free yogurt
¾ cup	Shredded carrot
½ cup	Mashed banana
1 tbs	Vanilla extract
¼ cup	Chopped pecans

Directions

Step 1: Mix the first 5 ingredients in a large bowl.

Step 2: Whisk oil, sugar and eggs in a moderate bowl. Yogurt and next adds 3 ingredients. In a large bowl, stir oil mixture into flour mixture. Stir in pecan nuts.

Step 3: Place a paper or foil liners in a 6-cup muffin pan. Divide batter evenly among muffin cups.

Step 4: Bake at 375° for 22 minutes or down to muffins are lightly browned and clean with a toothpick in center.

Lemony Hummus

Ingredients

2	Garlic cloves, peeled
1 can (15-ounces)	Chickpeas or garbanzo beans, rinsed and drained
¼ cup	Lemon juice
3 tbs	Water
2 tbs	Tahini
1 tbs	Ground cumin
¼ tbs	Salt
¼ tbs	Pepper
	Pita breads, warmed and cut into wedges
	Carrot and celery sticks

Directions

Step 1: Process garlic in a meal processor till minced. Add chickpeas, lemon juice, water, tahini, cumin, salt, and pepper. Cover and process until creamy. Pour into a small bowl. Dish with pita wedges and vegetables.

Chicken Tortilla Soup

Ingredients

1 (14.5-ounce) can	Can Mexican-style stewed tomatoes, undrained
2 ½ cups	Water
2 cups	Cooked chicken, shredded (about 10 ounces)
2 cups	Stir-fry vegetables (yellow, green, and red peppers and onions)
1 cup	Reduced sodium chicken broth
2	Cloves garlic, minced
1 cup	Bag tortilla chips
1	Sliced fresh jalapeño chile peppers (see Tip)

Directions

Step 1: Combine tomatoes, water, chicken, frozen vegetables, broth, and garlic in a 3 1/2- or 4-quart slow cooker. Cover and simmer on low heat for 6-7 hours or high heat for 3-3 1/2 hours (see tips).

Step 2: Top each serving with tortilla chips. Sprinkle chili pepper if you like.

Tips

Line the slow cooker with disposable slow cooker liners for easy cleanup. Add ingredients according to recipe. When you're done cooking your meal, simply spoon the food out of the slow cooker and discard the liner. Do not pick up or carry disposable bags containing food.

Chili peppers contain volatile oils that can burn your skin and eyes, so avoid direct contact as much as possible. Wear plastic or rubber gloves when handling chili peppers. If you touch peppers with your bare hands, wash your hands and nails thoroughly with soap and warm water.

Tomato and Basil Frittata

Ingredients

¼ cup	Diced onion I used sweet yellow onions
	Cooking spray
10	Eggs
½ cup	Milk I used 1%
1/23 tbs	Salt
¼ tbs	Black pepper
1 cup	Shredded part skim mozzarella divided
1 cup	Sliced tomatoes
10-15 leaves	Fresh basil

Directions

Step 1: Preheat your oven to 375.

Step 2: Add eggs, milk, salt and pepper to a medium bowl and mix well.

Step 3: Mix half of cheese into egg mixture and set aside.

Step 4: Spray a 10-inch nonstick skillet with cooking spray and heat over medium-high heat.

Step 5: Add the diced onions and cook until translucid, about 3 minutes.

Step 6: Put the tomato slices into the pan.

Step 7: Pour the egg mixture over the tomatoes and onions.

Step 8: Cook on stovetop over medium-low heat until edges begin to set, about 4 minutes.

Step 9: Use a spatula to loosen the edges and pull inwards to allow more of the egg to enter the hot pan.

Step 10: Repeat this several times. (I turned the pot about 3 times)

Step 11: Remove the pan from the heat.

Step 12: Top with basil leaves and sprinkle with the other half of the cheese.

Step 13: Place the pan in the oven until the center is set. Mine took 15 minutes.

Step 14: Remove the pan from the oven and let it cool slightly for about 5 minutes.

Step 15: If desired, use a spatula to transfer to a platter. (At this point you can give it a high five by using a non-stick coating!)

Step 16: Using a knife, cut the frittata into 8 pieces. Create giant plus signs (cut in quarters) and cut each of those pieces in half.

Step 17: Dish immediately. Leftovers can be stored in the refrigerator for up to 1 week.

Butternut Squash and Carrot Soup

Ingredients

1 tbs	Butter or margarine
3 cups	Peeled, diced butternut squash (about 1 small squash)
2 cups	Thinly sliced carrots (4 medium carrots)
¾ cup	Thinly sliced leeks or chopped onion
2 (14.5-ounce) cans	Reduced-sodium chicken broth
¼ tbs	Ground white pepper
¼ tbs	Nutmeg
¼ cup	Regular or fat-free half-and-half or light cream
1	Bunch Fresh tarragon leaves

Directions

Step 1: Heat a large saucepan over medium heat and melt the butter or margarine. Add squash, carrots, leeks or onions to pan. Cover and cook 8 minutes, stirring occasionally. Add broth. Bring to a boil. reduce heat. Cover and simmer 25 minutes or until vegetables are very tender.

Step 2: Place 1/3 of pumpkin mixture into the bowl of a food processor or blender jar. Cover; process or blend until nearly smooth. Repeat with remaining mixture. Return mixture to pan. Add white pepper and nutmeg. Just bring to a boil. Add half-and-half or light cream. heat up. Pour into soup bowl. Garnish with fresh tarragon if desired.

Grilled Shrimp Skewers

Ingredients

1-pound	Large shrimp peeled and deveined (you can either leave tails on or remove them)
¼ cup	Olive oil
2 tbs	Lemon juice
¾ tbs	Salt
¼ tbs	Pepper
1 tbs	Italian seasoning
2 tbs	Minced garlic
1 tbs	Chopped parsley
	Lemon wedges for serving

Directions

Step 1: Place olive oil, lemon juice, salt, pepper, Italian seasoning, and garlic in a zip lock bag. Cap and shake to mix.

Step 2: Place the shrimp in a bag and seal. Spread marinade evenly.

Step 3: Marinate for at least 15 minutes, or up to 2 hours. Do not marinate longer than this as the acid in the lemon juice will start to cook the shrimp.

Step 4: Skewer the shrimp. Heat a grill or grill pan over medium-high heat.

Step 5: Place skewers on grill. Fry 2-3 minutes per side or until shrimp is pink and opaque.

Step 6: Broiler Instructions: Preheat the grill. Arrange shrimp skewers on a baking sheet coated with cooking spray. Grill 2 to 3 minutes per side or until shrimp is pink and opaque.

Step 7: Sprinkle with parsley and garnish with lemon wedges.

CHAPTER TWELVE

RECIPES FOR GESTATIONAL DIABETES

Old-Fashioned Oatmeal

Ingredients

1 cup	Water or low-fat milk
pinch	Salt
½ cup	Rolled oats
2 tbs	Low-fat milk for serving
1 to 2 tbs	Honey, cane sugar or brown sugar for serving
pinch	Cinnamon

Directions

Step 1: Mix water (or milk) and salt in a small saucepan. bring to a boil. Stir in oatmeal and reduce heat to medium. Cook for 5 minutes, stirring occasionally. Remove from heat, cover and leave for 2-3 minutes.

Step 2: Top with milk, sweetener, cinnamon, dried fruit and nuts if desired.

Salmon Salad

Ingredients

½ cup	Boneless, skinless canned salmon, flaked (2 1/2 ounces)
1 tbs	Extra-virgin olive oil
1 tbs	Lemon juice
2	Kalamata olives, pitted and diced
1 tbs	Minced red onion, or to taste
1 tbs	Minced fresh parsley
1 tbs	Rinsed and chopped capers

Directions

Step 1: In a small bowl, combine salmon, oil, lemon juice, olives, red onion, parsley, and capers.

Zucchini Noodles with Quick Turkey Bolognese

Ingredients

3 cups	Quick Turkey Meat Sauce
8 cups	Zucchini noodles (from 3 medium zucchini)
½ cup	Grated Parmesan cheese

Directions

Step 1: Prepare Quick Turkey Meat Sauce by following the directions.

Step 2: While the sauce is cooking, divide the zucchini noodles into 4 covered serving containers (about 2 cups per container).

Step 3: Add 3/4 cup sauce and 2 tablespoons Parmesan cheese to each container. It can be sealed and stored in the refrigerator for 4 days.

Step 4: To reheat, remove lid and microwave on high for 2 1/2 to 3 minutes, until sauce is steaming and pasta is tender.

To make ahead: Store in refrigerator for up to 4 days.

Quick Turkey Meat Sauce

Ingredients

1 tbs	Extra-virgin olive oil
1	Large onion, chopped
4	Cloves garlic, minced
1 tbs	Italian seasoning
1-pound	Lean ground turkey
8-ounces	Mushrooms, chopped
½ tbs	Salt
1(28 ounce) can	Crushed tomatoes
½ cup	Chopped fresh parsley or basil

Directions

Step 1: Heat the oil in a large frying pan over medium heat. Add the onion and cook, stirring, until softened, about 5 minutes. Stir in garlic and Italian seasoning. Cook until fragrant, about 1 minute. Add turkey, mushrooms, and salt. Cook, crumble turkey with a wooden spoon and stir until turkey is no longer pink and mushrooms are cooked through, about 10 minutes.

Step 2: Increase warmness to medium-high. Stir in tomatoes and cook, stirring occasionally, till thickened, approximately five minutes. Stir in parsley (or basil).

Florentine Hash Skillet

Ingredients

1 tbs	Extra-virgin olive oil
½ cup	Frozen hash browns or precooked shredded potatoes (see Note)
½ cup	Frozen chopped spinach
1	Large egg
pinch	Salt
pinch	Freshly ground pepper
2 tbs	Shredded sharp Cheddar cheese

Directions

Step 1: Heat the oil in a small nonstick skillet over medium-high heat. Layer hash browns and spinach in skillet. Beat the eggs and sprinkle with salt, pepper and cheese. Cover and cook over medium-low heat, until hash browns begin to brown on the bottom, eggs are set, and cheese is melted, 4 to 7 minutes.

Tips:

Ingredient note: Shredded boiled potatoes can be found in the refrigerated or dairy section of most supermarkets.

Cherry, Wild Rice & Quinoa Salad

Ingredients

¾ cup	Wild rice
½ cup	Quinoa (see Tips), rinsed if necessary
¼ cup	Extra-virgin olive oil
¼ cup	Fruity vinegar, such as raspberry or pomegranate
¾ cup	Salt
¼ cup	Freshly ground pepper
2 cups	Halved pitted fresh sweet cherries (see Tips)
2 stalks	Celery, diced
¾ cup	Diced aged goat cheese, smoked Cheddar or other smoked cheese
½ cup	Chopped pecans, toasted (see Tips)

Directions

Step 1: Bring water to a boil in a large pot over high heat. Add wild rice and simmer for 30 minutes. Add the quinoa and simmer until the rice and quinoa are tender, about 15 minutes. Drain until cool to the touch and rinse with cold water. Drain well.

Step 2: Meanwhile, whisk together oil, vinegar, salt, and pepper in a large bowl. Add rice, quinoa, cherries, celery, cheese and pecans and mix. Serve at room temperature or chilled.

Tips:

Make Ahead Tip: Cover and refrigerate for as much as four hours.

Tips: Quinoa, a grain that was a staple food of the ancient Incas, was once only found in health food stores, but is now available in most major supermarkets and even warehouses. Residues of saponin, a protective coating, are removed. Most quinoa is sold already rinsed. Check the label.

To pierce fresh cherries, use a tool made for the job - hand-held cherries. It works for olives too! Alternatively, use the tip of a knife or peeler to pry the wick open.

Toast the chopped or sliced nuts in a small dry skillet over medium-high heat, stirring constantly, until fragrant and slightly browned, 2 to 4 minutes. Spread nuts whole on baking sheet and bake at 350°F, stirring once, until fragrant, 7 to 9 minutes.

Very Green Lentil Soup

Ingredients

2 tbs	Extra-virgin olive oil, plus more for garnish
2	Large yellow onions, chopped
1 ¼ tbs	Salt, divided
4 cups	Water, divided
1 cup	French green (Le Puy) or brown lentils
8	Large green chard leaves
1	Medium Yukon Gold potato, scrubbed
12 cups	Gently packed spinach (about 10 ounces), any tough stems trimmed
4	Scallions, cut into 1-inch pieces
5 cups	Vegetable broth, store-bought or homemade
2 cups	Chopped broccoli
1 tbs	Cumin seeds, lightly toasted and ground (see Tip)
½ tbs	Ground coriander
	Freshly ground pepper to taste
1 cup	Chopped fresh cilantro
2 tbs	Chopped fresh mint
½	Jalapeno pepper, minced
1 tbs	Fresh lemon juice, or more to taste
	Crumbled feta cheese for garnish

Directions

Step 1: Heat 2 tablespoons of oil in a large frying pan over high heat. Add onion and 1/4 teaspoon salt; Cook, stirring frequently, until onions begin to brown, about 5 minutes. Reduce the heat to low, add 2 tablespoons of water and cover. Cook, stirring frequently, until pan is cool, 25 to 35 minutes. Cover the pot from time to time and simmer until the onions are much reduced and caramelized.

Step 2: Meanwhile, rinse the lentils and pick a small stone. Combine lentils and remaining 4 cups water in a stockpot or Dutch oven. Turn off heat, reduce heat to low, cover and simmer for 20 minutes. Cut white ribs from chard. Chop vegetables, chop off ribs (keep in separate batches). Divide potatoes into 1/2-inch cubes. Chopped spinach; set aside.

Step 3: When the lentils are cooked for 20 minutes, stir in the chard ribs, potatoes, leeks, broth, and remaining teaspoon salt. Return to gentle simmering. Cover and cook for 15 minutes.

Step 4: Stir in chard leaves, broccoli, cumin, and coriander. Once the onions have caramelized, stir the broth slightly. Add them to the soup. Turnover, reduce heat, cover and simmer for another 5 minutes. Stir in reserved spinach, coriander, mint, jalapenos, and pepper. Reduce heat again, cover, and simmer until spinach is tender and still bright green, about 5 minutes. Stir in 1 tablespoon lemon juice. Taste and add lemon juice and pepper to taste. Serve each bowl of soup with olive oil and crushed feta cheese.

Tips

Tip: Toast the cumin in a skillet over medium-high heat, stirring occasionally, until fragrant, about 2 minutes. Cool slightly. Grind to a fine powder in a spice grinder, blender, or clean coffee grinder.

To make ahead: Cover and store in the refrigerator for up to 3 days.

Frozen Chocolate-Banana Bites

Ingredients

2	Medium bananas
1 ½ ounces	Special dark chocolate pieces (about 1/3 cup)

Directions

Step 1: Peel Bananas. Cut bananas into 1/2-inch thick slices. Line a baking sheet with parchment or wax paper. Arrange the banana pieces in a single layer on the prepared baking sheet.

Step 2: Melt the chocolate in a thick saucepan over low heat. Place the melted chocolate in a small resealable plastic bag. Seal the bag and cut off a small corner. Sprinkle chocolate over banana slices. Refrigerate for 1 to 2 hours or until frozen.

Step 3: Divide the banana pieces into 4 freezer containers or small resealable freezer bags. Freezes up to 3 days.

Veggie & Hummus Sandwich

Ingredients

2 slices	Whole-grain bread
3 tbs	Hummus
¼	Avocado, mashed
½ cup	Mixed salad greens
¼	Medium red bell pepper, sliced
¼ cup	Sliced cucumber
¼ cup	Shredded carrot

Directions

Step 1: Place hummus on one slice of bread and avocado on the other. Add vegetables, peppers, cucumbers, and carrots to sandwiches. Serve in half.

Guacamole-Stuffed Egg

Ingredients

6	Large eggs
1	Ripe avocado, diced
¼ cup	Prepared fresh tomato salsa
1 tbs	Lemon juice
	Kosher salt & cracked black pepper to taste

Directions

Step 1: Place the eggs in a single layer in the pan. Cover with water. Bring to a boil over medium heat. Reduce heat and simmer on low heat for 10 minutes. Remove from heat, drain, and cover eggs with ice water. Touch the water and let it sit until it cools before peeling. Cool to room temperature or refrigerate until cold.

Step 2: Meanwhile, in a medium bowl, mix avocado with salsa and lemon juice, but mash until still slightly clumpy.

Step 3: Halve each egg. Remove and discard the yolk. Top each half with 2 teaspoons of guacamole. Sprinkle with salt and pepper.

Tips

Make Ahead Tip: Cover unpeeled hard-boiled eggs and refrigerate for up to 1 week.

Roast Chicken with Parmesan-Herb Sauce

Ingredients

2	Bone-in, skinless chicken breasts (12 ounces each)
¾ tbs	Kosher salt, divided
½ tbs	Ground pepper, divided
3 tbs	All-purpose flour
4 tbs	Extra-virgin olive oil, divided
2	Bunches broccolini (8 ounces each)

3	Cloves garlic, minced, divided
1/3 cup	Dry white wine
1 cup	Low-sodium chicken broth
¼ cup	Grated Parmesan cheese
2 tbs	Chopped fresh thyme, divided
2 cups	Cooked whole-grain rice blend

Directions

Step 1: Place rack in lower third of oven. Preheat to 425 degrees Fahrenheit.

Step 2: Cut the chicken breast diagonally into 2 equal parts and sprinkle each with 1/4 teaspoon salt and pepper. Place the flour in a shallow bowl and lightly dredge the chicken. Set aside remaining flour. Heat 2 tablespoons oil in a large skillet over medium-high heat. Add the chicken, skin side down. Cook until bottom is browned, about 6 minutes. Place skin side up on a rimmed baking sheet. reserve the bread

Step 3: Toss the broccolini with the remaining 2 tablespoons oil, half the garlic cloves, and 1/4 teaspoon salt. Spread on the remaining half of the baking sheet.

Step 4: Cook until broccoli is tender and an instant-read thermometer inserted into thickest part of chicken registers 165 degrees Fahrenheit, 15 to 20 minutes.

Step 5: Meanwhile, combine 4 teaspoons of flour and wine in a small bowl and mix. Heat a frying pan over medium heat, add the remaining garlic, and heat for 30 seconds while stirring. Add broth. Bring to a boil over high heat. Add the wine mixture and cook, stirring frequently, until thickened and reduced to about 1 cup, 4 to 5 minutes. Add Parmesan cheese, 1 teaspoon thyme, and remaining ¼ teaspoon salt and pepper.

Step 6: To serve, divide chicken, broccoli and rice among 4 plates. Pour the sauce over the chicken and sprinkle with the remaining 1 teaspoon of thyme.

Tips:

Cut Down on Dishes: The rimmed baking sheet is great for everything from frying to catching accidental drips and spills. For hassle-free cleaning and keeping your baking tray in tip-top shape, line it with foil before use please.

Lime & Parmesan Popcorn

Ingredients

2 cups	Plain air-popped popcorn
	Olive oil cooking spray
1 tbs	Parmesan cheese
1 tbs	Lime zest
pinch	Chili powder
pinch	Salt

Directions

Step 1: Lightly coat the popcorn with cooking spray. Stir in Parmesan cheese, lime zest, chili powder, and salt.

CHAPTER THIRTEEN

CONCLUSION

Diabetes is a difficult disease for both children and parents. Physical, emotional and psychological stress are daily challenges for people with diabetes. The rate of newly diagnosed patients has increased exponentially over the years, and this is inexplicably done by doctors, but not by awareness and education. To do so, we must first raise awareness of diseases, conditions, treatments, management, complications, and prevention.

There are two forms of diabetes, type 1 and type 2. About 95% of diabetics have his type 2, but only 5% of Americans have her type 1. Type 2, sometimes called adult-onset diabetes, is more common than type 1, also known as "juvenile" diabetes, but is often considered the more serious of the two. Type 1 diabetes is most commonly diagnosed in children. However, it can be diagnosed in adulthood. When the body eats food, the stomach begins to break down the contents into proteins, fats, and carbohydrates. It is carbohydrates that are further broken down into glucose, which the body uses as energy. In a normal, healthy body, the pancreas releases a hormone called insulin that helps cells take up and use glucose. glucose is absorbed. But without insulin, cells cannot open up and absorb glucose from the bloodstream. The pancreas in people with type 1 diabetes does not function properly. It releases little or no hormone insulin. Therefore, once glucose enters the bloodstream, it has to stay there. Type 1 diabetes is considered an "autoimmune disease" because the insulin-producing beta cells of the pancreas attack the immune system early in the disease process. This is because it is attacked by and 'accidentally' destroyed, resulting in insufficient insulin production in the pancreas." Therefore, people with type 1 diabetes require insulin therapy to maintain normal blood sugar levels.

Diabetes is an autoimmune disease that scientists believe is genetically linked. Genes are "like instructions for how the body looks and functions...but just getting the genes for diabetes is usually not enough. Most of the time a person gets the type to do so, another thing has to happen, such as a viral infection.1 Diabetes. In other words, diabetes is not considered an infectious disease and is not like the common cold that you get from coming into contact with someone who has the disease.

9 798385 789375